Get your mind right to shake the weight off.

M.R. Temple

ISBN: 1502966859
ISBN-13: 978-1502966858

DEDICATION

These books dedicated to my beautiful family, but most of all, my wonderful wife, Josephine Richardson. Thank you for supporting me with your actions and not your words. When the mornings were cold and wet, you were right by my side rain or shine. When I was weak and wanted to go to the food dealer, you were my conscious. Last but not least, I'd like to thank life for posing the challenge.

CONTENTS

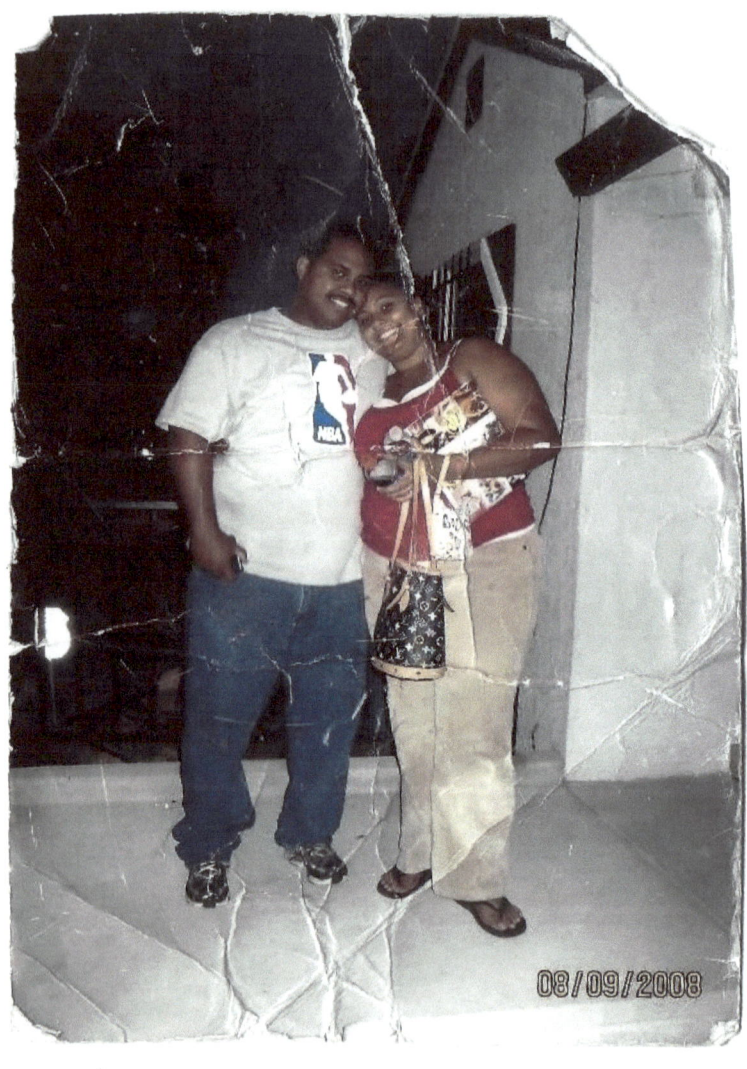

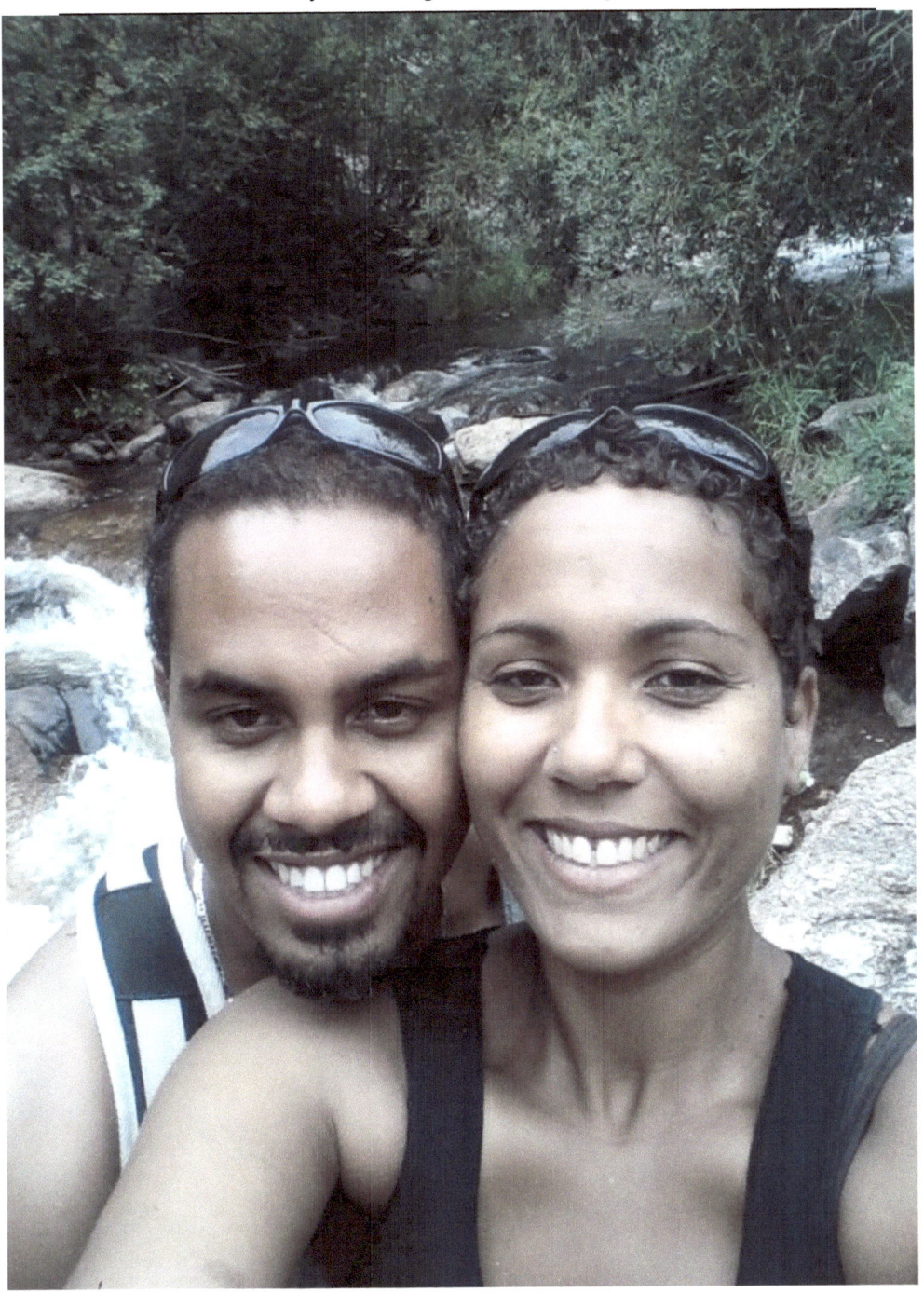

How I lost my weight

Who is this guy, and why do I have his book? In my opinion, I am nothing more than a typical American who, like a lot of

Americans, I was overweight. It's true - the sexy man that wrote this book once weighed over two hundred and eighty pounds, and my equally hot wife of eighteen years weighed in at 268 pounds.

I married my high school sweetheart, who I fell in love within

August 1996, and never looked back. I'm a parent of three children, who we have homeschooled ever since my oldest, who is now 14, was in 1st grade. My wife was a stay at home mom who was shooting out children one after another for me. Well, the first two were for me, after that my little girl was all her. My wife did everything she could to get her. Let's just say she got what she wanted, and I got what I didn't know I needed, my baby girl.

While my wife was shooting out children, I was working three jobs and doing whatever else I could for income. I was a school bus driver and a school liaison by the time I was 21. That job was very stressful because it required me to deliver letters to people who were not keeping better track of their children in public school.

So, you can imagine that was a fun job with lots of stress. Naturally, I gained weight. I hit it big when I became a correctional officer at age 22. As many officers told me when I graduated from my long, grueling 16-week life in the academy, "you hit the lottery."

They were right, but as they say 'more money, more problems.' We started to make more money than we ever had before, so we did what all young people in their 20's so - we spent it! We never thought to invest because we wanted to buy useless "things" and give our babies the best "stuff." So, I worked harder and longer hours to get more money, which in turn helped me gain more weight. Money worries were over, but my stress level was about to take a big leap along with my waist size.

I still didn't learn my lesson about stress and how to manage it, so I pushed onward in my efforts to make more money. By the time I was about 24, I had become a counselor for the prison I was working at in California. The name of the medical prison is N.A Chaderjian.

Trust me when I say that being a medical, mental lock-up prison guard/counselor did wonder for my mind, gut, and butt. I was sitting more and become even more stressed out. I took on my counselor position when I almost weighed a whopping 250 -260 lbs. After one and a half years of crazy 16 hour shifts and the 1-hour commute each way, I started to rack up weight, and it was no joke. I now weighed 288 pounds after only three years of the worst sleeping and eating habits of my life due to being a father of three and a police officer/counselor.

I am telling you all of this so you can see that I am not one of those people who was born skinny and stayed skinny, and now I am
telling you what to do.
I am like most Americans; I just lost the weight, unlike most
Americans. I am a 35-year-old father of three.
I happen to know a thing or two about stress. In other words, I am no different than you. I am a hard-working person who wants to enjoy his weekends with good food and good drinks. I had to change the way I viewed weight loss.

I realized that the changes needed to start in my head, by being 100% honest with myself in every aspect of my life. I know it's much harder to do than it sounds. I knew I had to make the change because, even at 288 pounds, I felt like I was a skinny guy trapped in a fat man's body. I needed to lose weight. Here is where I made the typical American move - I bought diet supplies. I purchased the most embarrassing diet pills of all time, and they should have been

illegal.

Stockholm's Syndrome and Your Fat

What is Stockholm's Syndrome?

Stockholm's syndrome or capture-bonding is a psychological phenomenon in which hostages express empathy and sympathy and have positive feelings toward their captors, sometimes to the point of defending and identifying with them.

You know that you've heard the excuses made by comedians and your friends that "You have to love yourself no matter how big you get. To some extent, they are correct. You have to love yourself enough to see that you are the cause of your imprisonment, and you love yourself enough to get out of your self-imposed confinement. You have to change your perception of your situation to change your reality. If you're overweight and you have no illness that causes the weight gain, you need to recognize that you are the cause of your fat imprisonment.

To get out of the obese prison, one must first recognize that they put themselves in the prison cell.

Once you realize that you are your captor, the next steps are up to you. All that is required to do is reach down into your pocket, remove the keys that open the jail cell door, and free yourself. Stop screaming from behind the door to someone that is not there. Stop telling the figment of your imagination that you want out of the cell when you're the person that put you in the cell.

If you're reading this book or any other book on weight loss, you are trying to break free from the hold of your captor, "Fat." That is the start.

There is no way to break out of your bonds and set yourself free if you don't search for a way out of them. We don't just figuratively lock ourselves up; we do, too. How many times have you refused to do an activity because of your weight?

Or maybe you're like my wife, and She was requested to get off a roller coaster ride due to her weight. Her weight that day controlled her physical body. In California, a famous restaurant was closed and forced to relocate due to someone that was overweight and could not fit through the doors of the restaurant.

Instead of seeing what she has done to herself by eating that kind of food, she tried to sue the burger shop and have them closed down. The business just moved locations and found a way to keep their livelihood going.

The person that tried to sue them was obese; she is a clear case of a person controlled by her captor, the "fat cells." Her fat cells told her these people were not being thoughtful and didn't make room for her and her excessive weight.

She felt that she should be able to enjoy the same foods and life as an active person, but she was in for a real reality check. Her body is in a figurative prison. She was not free at all! The worst part about this prison is that you are the only one that is keeping you in it. We have the keys to our cell and the prison door; you just have to want freedom more than that burger or any addiction for that matter. You have to want to take control of your life and set yourself free.

Try this small experiment, if you are twenty-five pounds overweight, get a twenty-five-pound dumbbell, and start walking around the gym for three hours with the twenty-five-pound weight.

What you'll get is a taste of what your heart is feeling, except your heart never puts the weights down.

Now try and lie to yourself and say that twenty-five pounds isn't very much extra weight on your heart. Your heart is the motor of your body and is pushing or pulling you up, down, left, right, and side to side. You should never carry long-term excess weight. It can damage your ligaments and muscles. You can experience the same effect if you walk around with dumbbells in your hands, you're making your heart carry more than it should. That's called working out, and that's done in the gym, not every second of your life. When you are overweight, you are working out twenty-four seven weight loss is that it is 100% all on you and needs to that too needs to be done correctly.

If you choose liposuction, pills, shakes, personal trainer, Px90, or any other form of weight loss, you have to make the appointment, pay for the supplies, go to the doctor, or go to the store to purchase these things. The point I am trying to make is that it takes action, no matter what route you choose. Positive reactions in the right step can and will help everybody get a step closer to being free from their captor "fat." One of the most freeing actions you can take is lacing your shoes up and walking every day for twenty minutes and drink as much water as possible, if not exclusively. By starting with those small steps, you will begin to see weight loss, but you must start with baby steps.

Baby steps are the best for any overweight person not to get burnt out and to stay excited about working out. We spent most of our time watching T.V shows if we were not cooking, we were watching food on T.V. If we were not cooking for ourselves, we were preparing food for our friends and families that expect you to have food or sweets in your house. It takes baby steps for everyone around you to get used to your new way of life

My diet

I tried everything from pills that block your body from absorbing the fat from the food you eat, so you don't have to stop being a fat glutinous pig. That's right, you read it right, you can still taste the nasty the pickle your liver, kill yourself fast food and even lose weight, and they are right to a degree.

I have come to call it 'shock treatment.' The best way for me to explain this pill to you is by Dawn. Yes, "Dawn soap." Do you know how it makes the grease run away when you put a drop in your dirty pots? Well, these pills work in a similar way. When you eat a big fat juicy grease burger, you take that little pill, and it stops your body from absorbing the grease, which now allows the oil to slip right out the back door, even when you don't want to.

What you end up with is an orange or grease color in your underwear, if you're lucky. If you're not lucky, you'll absorb more grease then your body can hold onto or absorb, and the next thing you know, you're slipping out of your chair and your pants, because it's grease slipping out of your behind! What can your sphincter muscles do against fat?

Then you have the diets that have you to eat nothing but meat. Not good!! That is how you end up with the worst poo. Your body is not supposed to eat so much meat. Think about it.

We are nothing more than creatures apart of the food chain.

Then, we decided that as the human race, we are above nature, and we can eat the way we want, as much as we want, and then get mad that we don't look as sleek and as strong as the lion that eats enormous portions of meat.

One significant fact is that we are the super-intelligent humans that didn't take into account. Lions weigh somewhere around 600 to 800 pounds.

A lion can go up to 4 days without eating, after a good kill. We usually sit in an air-conditioned office and drive ourselves in oversized vehicles everywhere. Still, somehow we get the feeling that we need as much meat as possible on a daily bases. Why?

Because this is when getting your mind right needs to come into play.

That's right, you heard me! Before you can lose any real weight, and keep it off, you will have to put your mind in a place that will allow it to accept your new way of life.

You will have to change the way you see things in your life. Your perception is going to have to change for your reality to change. If you want to, you will change your life. I first stumbled on my problem when I was about 288 pounds, and in my seventh year on the job.

About this time is when I realized I had to gain a positive perception of everything in my life. As usual, I was working an overtime shift (not by choice) just finishing some case notes on one of the inmates assigned to me when out of nowhere, I started thinking about him and his drug addiction. His addiction was no different than my addiction to the big fat juicy steak burrito that I was about to devour.

Now, some might think, 'what's wrong with that? Man's got to eat?' Well, here's the problem - I bought two of those massive burritos, and I was only four hours into my shift, and I was eating my second burrito. It wasn't my fault; the burrito smelled so good.

My food addiction was so bad I couldn't even make it the two-mile distance from the burrito truck to my job.

My drug of choice is food

I was unable to control my desire for the taste of the food. I was now what society likes to call a "Crack Head," but not for crack. I had it for something that I could get any time day or night. I even had it delivered to me. I was officially a "Food head." To gain control of my life, I decided to apply the lessons that I was just teaching the inmates to myself. First, I had to acknowledge the fact that I was no better than the last man in my office. I have my own addiction; it just isn't a big evil, publicly hated drug. It was for food.

All different sorts of food! Anything I say that I wanted, I bought it and ate it. I also had to realize that I had a significant lack of self-control. Right then and there, I decided to start working on me.

The first thing I did was admit to myself, "I had a problem. "At that moment, I looked down at my massive gut and my roach coach burrito sitting on my desk and realized I had been lying to myself.

Next, I put the food away and walked out of the room. I set an alarm clock so that I could eat when it was supposed to. I figured I went to public school, and I've been programmed to eat at scheduled times I just need to get back to the program.

It was easier than I thought to fall back into that routine, only this time I was going to be in control. I figured that if a man can control himself, he can deprive himself. So I made sure to deprive myself of things I knew I did not need, and in return, I proved to myself that I had self-control.

I learned to talk to myself and ask myself the same question I ask the inmates assigned to my caseload questions like, "Are you being honest with yourself? Was your answer to the question the truth? Then I would tell them, "their answer doesn't matter to me, because when you leave my office, I will still write what I want in your file because what I decide to write down is based on what I observe.

Your actions will tell me if you are changing or not." If you can be completely honest with yourself, your efforts will show everybody that you told yourself the truth. If you can't be honest with yourself, then you're just living a lie, and a lie is no way to live. So I didn't talk about anything to anybody. I needed only to do what I needed to do, and everybody around me will see just how serious I am about my life.

If you have a gut and you know that you're eating way too much food and not working out nearly enough, ask yourself, "Do I deserve the big fat juicy burrito?"

I was indeed working sixteen-hour days, and I was commuting two hours round trip, but all I did was sit on my butt all day. Like most Americans, I was devouring more calories than I was using. I wasn't working on a construction site like I did when I was 18 in my father's business. I was behaving like most Americans – eating and not working out. I had to change the way I looked at food and fast. One method that helped me improve was to write a food journal. Keep track of how you feel as you begin your journey.

When you don't fill as though you will make it, your notes will help you see how much time you have devoted to weight loss and how good the past days have been.

Try and remind yourself that you are eating to live, not living to eat.

Keeping a journal also helps you keep better track of your time. Track how much T.V you watched versus walking or doing

something proactive in your weight loss. Use part of this page to write the thought that comes to you when you are reading this. There is no time like the present to start making the necessary changes needed to reach your health goals.

When it comes to losing weight, the fight can only be fought by you and you alone. You hold the keys to your motor. The ability to start and stop your progress is entirely up to you.

Your body is no different than a car

I started looking at myself as a car. I said, "If I have a full tank of gas and don't need to fill up, I will not stop to spend an over-inflated amount of money for gas. I can wait. I'll fill up when I get to my home town, where I know the gas is better and cheaper." So I would eat at home when I needed to. Now, this was not easy, because my wife is a chief who was staying home and homeschooling our children, so she felt the need to create, and I was her taster.

Am I complaining? Yes, she tried to keep me fat! I had to be honest with her and tell her, "No, I was not hungry," and "I will try it tomorrow." Did it hurt her fillings? Yes, but does she love my firm Gluteus Maximus? Yes. I made it a point to eat her food first; then, after that, it was fruit and vegetables for the rest of the day until dinner.

The key is being honest with you. Knowing when to say enough is enough. Recognize the difference in eating Just because you can, and ask yourself if you should. You can put your hand in the fire, but should you. It may sound like I am saying starve, but that is not what I am saying. I am merely saying that if you have not or will not exert the amount of energy that you have eaten for the day, and then you are storing energy away in fat cells. Stored energy is fat that you have not converted into energy stored in fat reserves.

We all know that fat is for hard times, but when are you going to have a hard time with food when there is a form of food on every corner in most Westernized countries? So, it will take you to be honest with yourself. If you want it, you have to tell yourself the truth - I am overweight, and I want to change it. If you genuinely want to change, it will come from within you.

Only you control yourself and what goes into your mouth. You have to read and look at what you are putting in your mouth. Then, be honest with yourself. I know I can, but should I?

The more you resist junk food and work to make the mental changes needed, the more you will see the physical changes you want.

T.V is the Enemy

You're Visual Sensors React to Commercials!

I know you've heard this for years, but it's very accurate. According to a report written by Ingrid Lunden, a reporter for TechCrunch comes from paidContent.org, where she was a staff writer and has also written freelance articles for other publications such as the Financial Times. Ingrid covers mobile, digital media, advertising, and the spaces where these intersect.

According to Ingrid Lunden, research indicates that women spend almost forty minutes more than men watching straight television every day — four hours, eleven minutes for women; three hours thirty-four minutes for men — men are spending more than twice as much time as women using gaming consoles — precisely forty-eight minutes compared to twenty-two minutes each day.

Add that usage to TV time and the gap between how much time men and women spend in front of the screen narrows — although women are still ahead of men in TV screen time by a space of eleven minutes.

If we were to change our perception of the T.V., it's just a short Cyclops there to suck your time and thoughts away. I say thoughts because, like the teacher says, how can you be listening when you're talking? Well, how can you be thinking when you're watching, listening, and feeling emotional connections with a T.V. or movie character?

As for those that think you're thinking with the T.V on, wait until you see what you can do a few weeks after the crack/time-waster is no longer controlling your mind. When you take time from the T.V, you will find that T.V. keeps you in a state of excitement or drama and too much of anything is bad for you.

One way to tell if T.V is consuming your life is to see what your day to day thoughts and topics are when you're at work.

Do your thoughts consist of, 'Will they get off the island,' will finally get married?' Who cares? First, you have to ask why you should even care about what the in shape, hot, and sexy actors are doing at work. Don't forget that being hot and sexy on T.V is what they get paid to do. Focus on yourself and how you can become hot and sexy.

Actors have the luxury of being on the beach, shooting their shows or movies. They can afford a personal trainer to keep them on task, while you gain pound after pound, and New Year's resolution is broken shortly after New Year's resolution. How does it feel to continue to live your life on the couch while the T.V Cyclops sucks your youth, time, thoughts, and energy away just so that you can find out who is having sex with who and who was spotted where doing god knows what!

You need to be the sexy person getting spotted in wild places by your associates while you're in shape because you were able to get your mind right to shake the weight off.

When an actor needs to be motivated, they can afford to get a personal trainer to come to their house and push them. They also have their enormous paychecks that we provide by staying fat and devoting more time to T.V. than to our very own lives.

You have to change the way you see your time. How much of your time is spent in the sun with sweat on your skin, causing goosebumps to run down your spine right in the small of your back just as you come to a stop after you go for and complete a jog or walk? I found walking to be my number one way of losing weight. It was easier to walk than it was to jog at 288 pounds.

After my weight started to shake off

At this point and time of my life, I was super honest with myself about all of the foods I put in my mouth and what I allowed into my home. I kept focused on the fact that you are a product of your environment, so I made sure to keep my environment a healthy one.

By creating a clean, healthy space in my home, it helped keep my mind fresh and healthy. It made it easier for me to drop pounds fast, so fast that I felt like I need to go to the doctor to make sure I wasn't sick. After all, I worked in a medical, mental prison. As a counselor, I spent lots of time with people that have different types of severe illnesses that are highly contagious.

It was just one of the many dangers to the job, along with being attacked, killed, or having my family stocked by an angry parolee.

But to my relief, I was just losing a significant amount of weight from my life change. I cut out T.V. entirely for eight months. I still ate fast food, so to say I didn't eat the most addictive drug on the planet would be a lie and hypocritical. I ate just the burger from the fast-food chains. But then the time came when I had to have another heart to heart with myself again and this time get even more honest with me. I had to stop eating the garbage altogether. I promised myself that I would only eat homemade food and fresh fruits and vegetables.

After the" let's stop lying to myself talk I gave myself over and over again," I decided it was time to get myself educated on how to stay in shape so that when I come close to falling off of the wagon. I want to go back to the crack world, and I equipped myself with enough knowledge to battle the craving that just the smell of fast food brings to me. I had to be armed and ready to fight those feelings of happiness that come with giving into my addiction.

I started building my armory of weapons by not watching but studying one of the documentaries called "Fast *Food Nation"* and *"Supersize Me."* After that, I made a short journey down the road to *Food Matters*, while stopping off for the occasional episode of *You Are What You Eat*.

These were shows that kept me focused on not slipping back into bad habits. By staying focused on being honest with what I want for my life, I now fit into clothes I didn't know existed.

That was motivation enough to keep losing weight.

One day I wanted to show my wife just how much weight I lost. I put on her pants, and I showed her that I had lots of room in her pants. I have to say that that was the moment that made my wife sit down in front of the mirror and have the one on one she needed with herself.

My wife found as I did that when she placed herself in front of the mirror, she noticed in her reflection that she had her soda in her hand as usual. It hit her that Soda was her drug of choice, or her crack if you will. Reflecting on the drink caused her to realize she was killing herself, just like her father was. His drug of choice was alcohol, which caused him to leave his only daughter at a very young age. Believe me, if you get your mind right and you are truly honest with yourself, you, too, can look like the hot and sexy time stealing actors.

Change how you use your time

Look at the time in what I like to call your estimated life span. We hope that we can live happy 70-90 years. But in those 70-90 years, how much would it hurt you, if for the next six months or even six years of your remaining time you eat healthily? What if you only took six months just to drink water? What would be the worst-case scenario if you promised your body that you were not going to eat grease, fat, fake food, or unhealthy high fructose corn syrup for my source of energy?

If you take six months to drink only water, you will have plenty of time to go back to your old ways and do whatever you want to your body. I have to say, after being in great shape to being out of shape to being back in great shape, "There is nothing sweeter than being thin." If you look at your day-to-day and your week-to-week with the intent to make time, you will find a significant amount of time dedicated to things that could be replaced or moved around for about six months so you can invest in your body and mind. You cannot fix the body if you don't fix the brain. Time is never-ending, and you can't control it, just learn to manage it.

What I mean by that is there will always be something there to take up your time, but it is up to you to put things in priority of what needs to come first.

Your health or the late-night runs to the local pub or fast food joint? Use that time for just six months out of your 70-90 year life span to do some pushups, watch a documentary that will remind you why you don't eat that way, read a book, or write down the reasons why you think you put on so much weight. You have to learn to talk to yourself and ask real questions that only you know the answer. The time you spend for six months just walking and thinking and talking with a partner or friend will feel like the life you're living is so much better than the old one that you won't want to go back too.

I promise.

You will also find that by being knockdown, drag-out honest with yourself, there were a lot more things causing your weight gain than just T.V.

.

Monster Work Out

This portion of the book is perfect for everyone but is focused more on the dads than the moms. Playing Monster was my first form of exercise. After the T.V. went off, I realized my eleven, nine, and seven-year-old children were bored out of their minds, so I decided to give them a taste of my childhood. We went to the local park, and I became the monster that had to chase the children and devour them. They loved it. It not only gave me more endurance to play with my kids; it also gave me more energy in the bedroom to chase my wife down.

I would climb up the ladder on the jungle gym and run across the bridge, then slide down the firemen's pole. It was exhausting work.

The children understood daddy needed a few breaks to keep up the effort I was putting out. The laughter of my children drove me to want to work harder, so I will be able to hike and run after my grandkids someday. I remember asking my wife, "How long do you think you could run after the guy who takes your kid?" We both thought about it and realized we needed to change. But we didn't. That was at about 135 pounds on my way to 288. So, now I pose the question to you.

How long do you think you could run after your child if they are snatched in front of you?

What is exercise? One dictionary gave me these answers. NOUN:

• An act of employing or putting into play; use: the free exercise of intellect; the exercise of an option.

• Activity that requires physical or mental exertion, primarily when performed to develop or maintain fitness: took an hour of vigorous daily exercise at a gym.

A task, problem, or other effort performed to develop or maintain fitness or increase skill: a piano exercise; a memory exercise.

You can see how exercising your mind and body is needed to stay balanced. You have to make help mind remember your goals and expectations. You can't let it tell your body, 'I can rest today.' Not if you know that you have not earned the rest. Be honest with yourself. It is exhausting but worth it.

How horrible would it be if what stood between you and your child's safety was a large gut caused by a few cheeseburgers or tacos? If someone snatched your child in front of you at the park, could you run long enough to apprehend the kidnapper, or would they getaway? Could you run fast enough, hard enough, and long enough to catch the criminal?

It only takes 30 minutes a day to build a long-lasting relationship with your kids at the park, and you gain physical endurance. Never mind that you are teaching them to take their health seriously, and you are teaching them how to be an excellent interactive parent for the future when they become worn out exhausted parents.

The more you play, the more your body gets used to running and jumping. Your brain loves oxygen, and your actions will build excellent muscle memory. Another plus is that your children are always up for a day, or even an hour, at the park.

Crazy Apples

I titled this chapter Crazy Apples because this is one of my favorite workouts. Try and make eating an apple or two for breakfast a routine, then put on your favorite jams and just let loose. Now, be very honest with yourself - are you dancing as hard as you could, or are you embarrassed by what people think of you, even yourself? I would put on my absolute favorite music and lose it. I looked like Kevin Bacon from the movie *Footloose*. What I found was that I was losing weight just because I was moving my body. I was not only letting my energy stay stored in my stomach and legs.

All of the fruits and vegetables I had been eating acted like high octane gas in my tank. It made me want to keep eating fruits and vegetables throughout the day and, of course, other things like peanut butter and honey on wheat.

I did this workout in the morning about four times a week (you need some time to rest). By creating a movement routine, you're using the stored energy in your fat cells. If you stop and do 5 to 10 pushups three times a day, you will see a significant difference in your chest, arms, and back after about two weeks.

So, after six months of just dancing to your favorite music and cutting out the extra fat in your life, you will lose lots of weight.

Write down your food plan for each day.

1.

2.

3.

4.

5.

6.

7.

8.

9.

10.

Eat breakfast

Believe it or not, eating breakfast is better than not eating breakfast at all; some breakfast options are better than others. Getting the right combination of nutrients will help you feel full of energy and just plain full until lunch, while eating the wrong foods for breakfast may have you reaching for a doughnut or other less healthy snack option a short time later.

The fruit is one of the components of a healthy breakfast because it provides vitamins, minerals, water, and fiber. Fiber helps to slow down the digestive process and keep you full longer. The vitamins and minerals help you meet your daily requirements for these nutrients, which is hard to do if you skip breakfast. Oatmeal with fruit and milk, yogurt with fruit and granola, a fruit smoothie with toast and peanut butter, and fruit juice with a breakfast burrito made with a whole grain tortilla all make delicious and nutritious options for breakfast.

You can stock up on portable breakfast options to make it easier to fit this meal into your days, such as fruits that are easy to carry with you, granola bars, and cups of yogurt.

Crazy Apples are more than just apples; it's about all kinds of fruits that get you moving and staying moving for as long as your favorite song can touch you. Since the beginning of time, humans and music have gone hand in hand.

Music takes your mind off physical pain, sorrow, and time. You can listen to a whole CD and not realize you just spent two hours listing to your favorite jam, and the most you did was bob your head. If you love it, dance, move, burn fat, and feel tired.

The more you move, the more you burn. The more you burn, the smaller your pant or dress size will get. The other fantastic quality that Crazy Apples adds to your life is that if you do have a real job, you will have added more cardio to your daily workout. That, in turn, means you will burn twice as much fat in one day. The more you burn, the more fat, transformed from storage into energy for your body. Soon you will be losing lots and lots of fat all over your body.

You will notice that your neck has shrunk, you've reunited with your feet and other parts that have gone missing.

When you have reached your weight loss goal, you get to increase your intake because you have burned more than you needed for the day. That is what I call a surplus. You have saved enough space to put some fat back into the bank. Feel free to have that nice dinner at the restaurant and the extra drink that day. But be sure to take it day by day, not week by week. After all, yesterday and tomorrow don't genuinely exist, only now does.

So if you mess up, it is ok. Just fix it immediately and don't wait until tomorrow because tomorrow doesn't exist. Fruits and vegetables are a vital source of vitamins, minerals, and fiber that support a healthy body and prevent serious illnesses.

A diet rich in fruits and vegetables helps us maintain healthy, happy well-being, and it also is a primary fighter in helping the body combat stress.

Just Water for 6 Months

It is only six months out of your entire nitty-year life span. Really, how much is that? All I am asking is that you suck down water for six months to see how your body reacts to it. Your skin will clear up, your body will thank you with better bowel movements, and your organs will just plain feel better, and it only takes a few months out of your ninety-year life span. What is stopping you from devoting a little bit of time to your body's wellbeing? We have no problem with eating spicy stuff when we shouldn't or drinking too many nights in a row.

We will ask so much from our body but give it so little. We think we are giving it good stuff, but do you take it for a walk like your dog needs? Do you feed it like your dog is supposed to be feed?

Do you treat other's lives better than your own life? Pretend your mind is separate from your body. Your brain may sleep great, and you may be smart as a whip, but if the body's neglected, your body will die.

So your body will die, but your mind will feel energetic. The computer will function, but without its shell to protect it from destructive particles, it will die, so will your brain. Water is the most important thing your body can have. It cleans all your organs, along with the largest one of all, your skin. You sweat all the time when you work out and drink water. Water is the most critical substance and the most abundant substance in the human body. Water comprises about three-quarters of the human mass and is a significant component of every cell. Water is also essential for removing toxins from the human body.

The body removes toxins in many ways bowels, urination, and sweat. These methods directly excrete water from the body. When dehydrated, the body will try to save water by minimizing the use of the first three functions and will force the liver to assume as much of the workload as possible. This extra work will place a heavy burden on the liver, which has other functions in addition to detoxification. Even then, the organ

(Liver) by itself will not be able to do all the work very efficiently, and toxins will build up rapidly.

Water is also crucial to fitness and fat loss for several reasons, including the following: Water fills us up without adding any calories.

Dehydration will degrade a person's ability to exercise and burn calories. Dehydration will reduce protein synthesis, which is needed to build and repair muscles.

It's recommended to drink about two to three quarts of water per day. However, this will vary with the size and activity level of the person, as well as with climate conditions. Either case, if your urine is bright yellow, then you need to drink more water. Also, anyone who exercises nonstop for more than an hour should consider replacing electrolytes along with the water. This is to avoid hypernatremia (depleted sodium) or other forms of severe electrolyte depletion, which can be dangerous. Water is so essential that without it, YOU WILL DIE!

Life Change

This chapter has been titled " Life Change because a diet is something you do when you want to fit into something for a weekend, not something you do for life. You have to make changes that will come over time. They will become part of your everyday routine, and your friends will even learn to accept whatever method you have to keep you healthy and in shape.

Your spouse will encourage your workout, and your friends will either be jealous or support you. No matter what happens, you have to find joy in working out and in yourself.

Exercise programs need to change to be something you enjoy and keep apart of your life. That is why it is so crucial for you to change your perception so your perception can change your reality. By doing these things, you can get your mind right and not just accomplish weight loss but anything.

Once you make whatever routine that works for your work, you will feel powerful enough to take on the world. Once you combat your fat demon and win, you will defiantly feel ready for any battle in your life. You must find something that works. There are too many forms of exercise, such as walking, running, jogging, swimming, hiking, canoeing, kayaking, dancing, weight lifting, bike riding, rock climbing, and many, many more. That was just off the top of my head. You have to think, was there anything you liked doing when you were a kid that could make you lose weight. My wife took fencing classes. Which let me tell you, it takes more skill and muscle control then you would ever think.

Try out something new. Losing weight is about more than fitting in clothes and being liked by the people around you. Even when you're not fat anymore, they will find another reason to dislike you, so you have to want to change for you for at least six months out of your life, but start now. Nothing is stopping you from feeling like me except yourself. Break free of the prison you have placed yourself in and become more powerful than you have ever felt before. I've had my weight off for seven years now, and I am working on my sculpting.

Make life changes by getting your mind right. The rest will follow. After all, the body only goes where the head allows it to go.

You can now prepare to decide to put down the book and decide to continue down the path of obesity and body odors, or you decided this book was worth your time and start making life changes.

The only way to show it was worth your time is through your actions, so get up, put on your shoes, and start the first of many new days in your new life. You and only you have the power to change you!

If you noticed, this book is small, and the reason for that is because you need to spend your time walking and exercising, not reading a novel on how to lose fat.

ABOUT THE AUTHOR

I was born in Sacramento, California, in 1979. I married my high school sweetheart three years after dating. I supported my family at age 19 by becoming a school bus driver. Two years later, I took on a new position for the school district supervising seven schools. I assisted the principals by keeping the school up to date on the local gang's graffiti and truancy/after school fights.

Two years later, I took on the department of corrections medical, the mental institution when I was 22 years old. I worked in many different positions and many different areas of prisons for eight years. After quitting the prison, I moved to Colorado and followed the true passion I began writing.

I now have three books, two of which are online, and the third will one day be a movie. Look for my other books-

Cars and guns, what the difference? and

Rise of the W.I.T.C.H.E.S

Women in Touch Can Heal Every Soul